TONSILLITIS

Accurate Diagnosis, Effective Treatment, and Maintaining Respiratory Health: The Tonsillitis Handbook

CHAD BRUNO

Table of Contents

Introductory

Inflammation of the tonsils, two oval-shaped structures on either side of the back of the throat, is known as tonsillitis. Sore throat, difficulty swallowing, swollen tonsils, fever, and, occasionally, white or yellow patches on the tonsils are common signs of this illness, which can be caused by either a viral or bacterial infection. The painful and distressing symptoms of tonsillitis are frequently experienced, especially by children.

Tonsillitis can be either acute or chronic.

• The common cold virus and the Epstein-Barr virus (which causes infectious mononucleosis) are two examples of viruses that can cause tonsillitis. With rest and supportive care, viral tonsillitis usually resolves on its own.

• Tonsillitis caused by bacteria is called bacterial tonsillitis, and it is often caused by Streptococcus bacteria, hence the name "strep throat." Antibiotics may be necessary to treat bacterial tonsillitis and prevent complications like rheumatic fever.

Symptoms of tonsillitis range from a painful throat and fever to swollen and red tonsils, difficulty swallowing, and even enlarged lymph nodes in the neck. If tonsillitis is recurrent or severe, or if it leads to complications like abscess formation, chronic tonsillitis, or difficulty breathing and swallowing, a doctor may recommend treatment options, which can include antibiotics, pain relievers, and in some cases, surgical removal of the tonsils (tonsillectomy). The frequency and severity of tonsillitis bouts, among other considerations, are usually taken into account while deciding whether or not to remove the tonsils.

CHAPTER ONE
Tonsillitis Subtypes

Viral tonsillitis and bacterial tonsillitis are the two main categories of tonsillitis based on the etiology of the inflammation. Informed treatment decisions depend on correct categorization of these conditions.

1. Infectious tonsillitis:

• Virus-caused tonsillitis is the norm rather than the exception.

• Several viruses, including those that cause the common cold (such rhinovirus and adenovirus) and the flu, as well as the Epstein-Barr virus

(EBV), which causes infectious mononucleosis (mono), are to blame.

Sore throat, throat irritation, swallowing pain, mild to moderate fever, and other cold-like symptoms are common viral tonsillitis symptoms.

Treatment for viral tonsillitis consists mostly of rest, keeping hydrated, and using over-the-counter pain medicines to deal with discomfort; the condition usually clears up on its own within a week or two.

2. Strep throat, or bacterial tonsillitis:

• Group A Streptococcus (Streptococcus pyogenes) is the most prevalent bacterial cause of strep throat (bacterial tonsillitis).

• Symptoms of bacterial tonsillitis tend to be more severe than viral tonsillitis and might include a very sore throat, high fever, swollen and red tonsils with white or yellow spots, headache, and often swollen lymph nodes in the neck.

Antibiotics, mainly penicillin or amoxicillin, are used to treat strep throat and prevent its possible consequences, such as rheumatic fever. Antibiotics are crucial for reducing the severity of an infection, stopping its spread, and decreasing the likelihood of consequences.

Bacterial tonsillitis requires prompt antibiotic therapy since unchecked strep throat can develop to more serious complications.

Fungal tonsillitis, which typically affects those with weakened immune systems, and chronic or recurrent tonsillitis, which can occur from repeated episodes of either viral or bacterial tonsillitis, are also possible causes of tonsillitis. Seek medical attention if you feel you have tonsillitis or a throat infection, as the kind and source of your infection may affect the treatment options available to you.

Why Tonsillitis Occurs

Infections, typically viral or bacterial, are the main culprits in cases of tonsillitis. Tonsillitis is typically brought on by one of the following:

1. Illnesses Caused by Viruses: a. The common cold and viral tonsillitis are both caused by rhinoviruses, the virus responsible for the common cold. b. Tonsillitis is one of many respiratory illnesses caused by adenoviruses. c. Inflammation of the tonsils is a common symptom of infection with the influenza virus, sometimes known as the flu. d. The Epstein-Barr virus (EBV) is the causative agent of infectious mononucleosis (often known as "mono"), which can manifest clinically as acute tonsillitis.

2. Infectious Bacterial Diseases: a. Bacteria belonging to the group A Streptococcus (Streptococcus pyogenes) are the leading cause of strep throat and tonsillitis. Strep throat is a major health risk since it can develop into rheumatic fever if not addressed. b. Bacterial tonsillitis can also be caused by different bacterial pathogens, including but not limited to Group C and Group G Streptococcus and other bacteria.

The following are some other causes or aggravators of tonsillitis:

1. Tonsillitis is easily transferred by intimate contact with an infected person, which can be problematic in settings where there is a significant concentration of people, such as classrooms and homes.

2. People whose immune systems are already impaired may be at greater risk for developing tonsillitis and other problems.

3. Inflammation and irritation of the throat caused by allergies might increase the risk of infection in the tonsils.

4. Pollution and smoking, for example, are two environmental irritants that can aggravate throat irritation and increase the likelihood of developing tonsillitis.

Although infections are the most prevalent cause of tonsillitis, it is crucial to remember that certain people may experience chronic or recurring tonsillitis due to several episodes of infection. If tonsillitis persists for an extended period of time, a tonsillectomy (the surgical removal of the tonsils) may be considered. Sore throat, fever, and swallowing difficulties are all signs that you may have tonsillitis and should see a doctor to get a proper diagnosis and treatment plan.

CHAPTER TWO
Recognizing Tonsillitis Symptoms

It's crucial to get medical attention while experiencing symptoms of tonsillitis. The symptoms of tonsillitis, which can be brought on by either a viral or bacterial infection, can range in intensity. Tonsillitis typically manifests with the following symptoms:

1. The most common symptom of tonsillitis is a painful throat, which can range from moderate to severe.

2. Pain When Swallowing: If you have tonsillitis, you may have pain when trying to swallow, especially when eating solid foods.

3. The tonsils, which are in the back of the throat, might swell and turn red. They can grow so huge that they block the airway in extreme circumstances.

4. Tonsillitis caused by bacteria, such as strep throat, can cause white or yellow spots or streaks to appear.

5. Fever: Tonsillitis can be accompanied with a fever. Depending on how severe the infection is, the fever could be mild or severe.

6. Many people with tonsillitis also suffer from headaches, which can be related to the pain and swelling in the throat that comes with the infection.

7. Swallowing Difficulties: A sore throat and swollen tonsils can make swallowing uncomfortable and even painful.

8. Depending on the severity of the infection, the lymph nodes in the neck may swell and become tender.

9. Some people with tonsillitis have voice changes, such as hoarseness or a scratchy quality to their voice.

10. Tonsillitis can also bring on a chronic cough from postnasal drip or throat discomfort.

11. Tiredness or weariness is a common complaint among those suffering with viral tonsillitis.

12. Halitosis (Bad Breath): Pus or debris on the tonsils can cause bad breath from tonsillitis.

Tonsillitis can have a variety of symptoms, some mild and others severe, depending on whether it was caused by bacteria or viruses. Bacterial tonsillitis, especially strep throat, requires immediate treatment with medicines to prevent complications, whereas viral tonsillitis often cures on its own with rest and supportive care.

The best course of action if you or a loved one is experiencing these symptoms is to consult a doctor for an accurate diagnosis and treatment. Tonsillitis can be diagnosed by a doctor with the help of diagnostic tests like a throat swab, and the doctor can then prescribe antibiotics or other treatments to alleviate the symptoms.

Alternative Treatments

Tonsillitis treatment depends on the type of bacteria or virus causing the infection and the severity of the symptoms.

1. Care for Viral Tonsillitis with Supportive Measures:

If you want to help your body fight off the virus, the best thing you can do is relax.

Soothe your throat by staying hydrated with fluids like water, herbal teas, and clear soups.

A sore throat can feel better after gargling with warm saltwater.

An in-room humidifier can help alleviate sore throat symptoms by adding moisture to the air.

2. Viral or bacterial pain relief medication:

Nonprescription pain medicines, such as acetaminophen (Tylenol) or ibuprofen (Advil, Motrin), might alleviate discomfort and lower body temperature and inflammation. Be sure to strictly adhere to the recommended dosage.

3. Strep throat (bacterial tonsillitis) antibiotics:

Tonsillitis caused by Streptococcus bacteria (strep throat) will require antibiotic treatment from your doctor. Penicillin and amoxicillin are two of the most widely used antibiotics.

If you want to make sure the infection is entirely gone, it's important to take all of the antibiotics even if you start to feel better.

4. Surgical Extraction of the Tonsils (Tonsillectomy):

Tonsillectomy, the surgical removal of the tonsils, may be an option for people with chronic or severe tonsillitis.

When tonsillitis is severe enough to cause complications including abscess formation, obstructive sleep apnea, or trouble breathing and swallowing, a tonsillectomy may be recommended.

5. You should stay away from irritants, like:

Avoid environmental irritants such as secondhand smoke and smoking, as these can increase throat inflammation.

6. Steroids:

To alleviate pain and swelling in the throat, your doctor may recommend corticosteroids.

It's crucial to stick to the treatment plan prescribed by your doctor. Tonsillitis, and especially strep throat, is a serious condition that requires medical attention for diagnosis and treatment. Streptococcus pharyngitis can cause rheumatic fever if left untreated.

If you or your kid needs to have your tonsils removed, be sure to carefully adhere to all postoperative care recommendations, including those related to pain management and food restrictions.

Remember that tonsillitis is contagious, and good hygiene habits like frequent handwashing and avoiding close contact with infected individuals can help prevent its spread.

CHAPTER THREE
Treatment of Bacterial Tonsillitis with Antibiotics

Antibiotics are commonly used to treat bacterial tonsillitis, especially strep throat, because they are highly successful at curing the illness and preventing complications. Antibiotics for bacterial tonsillitis are typically recommended from the following groups:

1. **Penicillin:** Penicillin is frequently the first-line treatment for strep throat. Strep throat is typically caused by Group A

Streptococcus, which this remedy is effective against.

2. Antibiotics like amoxicillin, a penicillin derivative, are also frequently recommended for bacterial tonsillitis and strep throat. Its spectrum of activity is comparable to that of penicillin.

3. Penicillin allergy or resistance may lead to the prescription of other antibiotics.

• Penicillin-like cephalosporins (e.g., cephalexin, cefuroxime)

Azithromycin, Clarithromycin, and Other Macrolide Antibiotics

A. Clindamycin

Even if you feel better before the full course of antibiotics has been taken, it is still vital to take them as instructed by your doctor. Completing the full course of antibiotics is essential for killing out any remaining bacteria and preventing antibiotic resistance.

Here are some broad recommendations for treating bacterial tonsillitis with antibiotics:

• Follow the suggested dosage and time frame for taking the medication.

• Antibiotics are not to be shared, as each person's dosage and antibiotic of choice should be based on their unique infection.

Do not take two doses at once to make up for a forgotten one; rather, take the missed dose as soon as you remember but no more than two hours later.

If you have any adverse effects or allergic reactions, please inform your doctor immediately.

• It's possible that your symptoms won't improve right away, even if you begin antibiotic treatment. The drug may take a day or two to start working, and it may take several days to completely relieve symptoms.

To speed up your healing, be sure to drink plenty of water and get plenty of rest.

It is crucial to consult a doctor if you think you have bacterial tonsillitis or strep throat so that you can get a proper diagnosis and the right medications. Streptococcus pneumoniae can cause serious problems if left untreated.

Keeping Your Tonsils Healthy

Because many of the viruses that cause tonsillitis are very contagious and can be easily spread through close contact, prevention of tonsillitis, especially viral tonsillitis, can be difficult. Tonsillitis can be avoided, or at least its progress slowed, by following a few simple rules of hygiene and healthy living.

1. Hygiene of the Hands: Regular hand washing is one of the best strategies to stop the spread of germs that can lead to tonsillitis. Avoid spreading germs by not washing your hands thoroughly with soap and water after using the restroom or coming into close contact with someone who is ill.

2. Stay Away from Sick People It's best to stay away from sick people, especially if they have a sore throat or tonsillitis symptoms.

3. Avoid spreading potentially infectious respiratory droplets by protecting others from your coughs and sneezes by covering them with a tissue or your elbow. Don't forget to flush tissues and scrub your hands after using them.

4. Do not share utensils, glasses, or other personal belongings with people who are ill or who may be a carrier of an infectious disease.

5. Brush your teeth twice a day and rinse with mouthwash to keep your mouth healthy. This can help lessen the likelihood that tonsillitis will be brought on by a secondary bacterial infection.

6. Maintaining good health is important for fighting off infections. Eat well, exercise frequently, get plenty of sleep, and learn to cope with stress if you want a stronger immune system.

7. Avoid Smoking: Both active and passive smoking irritate the throat and tonsils, increasing the risk of infection.

8. Avoid direct contact with sick people and be particularly careful with your personal hygiene during cold and flu season.

9. The best way to prevent tonsillitis, which can be caused by a virus, is to be vaccinated. Tonsillitis caused by the flu virus is something that can be avoided by taking preventative measures, such as getting vaccinated.

10. You or a member of your household should get medical attention right once if you develop tonsillitis symptoms. Infections are less likely to spread if they are detected and treated quickly.

However, in instances where direct contact with sick individuals is difficult to avoid, even these precautions may not ensure complete prevention of tonsillitis. You or someone you know should see a doctor for a diagnosis and treatment plan if tonsillitis symptoms appear.

CHAPTER FOUR
Improving One's Immunity

Tonsillitis is a common infection that can be avoided by taking steps to boost your immune system. There is no magic bullet when it comes to maintaining a strong immune system, but there are a number of approaches you may take:

1. Maintain a Healthy Weight:

Eat a wide variety of fruits and vegetables to acquire the vitamins, minerals, and antioxidants your body needs to fight off illness. Vitamin D (found in fortified dairy products and fatty fish) and vitamin

C (found in citrus fruits) rich foods may have additional health benefits.

2. Avoid dehydration:

Take in enough of fluids to maintain your body's hydration levels. All biological processes, including the immune system, depend on adequate water intake.

3. Rest Your Brain:

Try to get between 7 and 9 hours of sleep every night. Getting enough shut-eye is crucial for maintaining a healthy immune system.

4. Stress Management:

The immune system can be compromised by prolonged stress. Try some stress-relieving activities like yoga, deep breathing, meditation, or just going outside for a while.

5. Get some regular exercise:

Regular moderate exercise can improve immunity. Exercise at least 150 minutes each week, preferably at a moderate level.

6. Keep Your Weight Down:

The immune system can be weakened by excess weight. The

immune system can benefit from a person achieving and maintaining a healthy weight through proper nutrition and exercise.

7. Take Care of Your Hygiene:

To stop the spread of disease, it's important to regularly wash your hands with soap and water. Don't put your dirty hands anywhere near your face.

8. Don't Overindulge or Smoke:

The immune system is weakened by smoking and drinking excessively. Quitting smoking and restricting alcohol intake can have a good impact on your health.

9. Immunity from vaccines can protect against contracting or transmitting some infectious diseases.

10. Maintain a Regular Immunization Schedule:

• Be sure you and your loved ones have all of your immunizations, including yearly flu shots and any other vaccines your doctor recommends.

11. Probiotics, Eat Them!

• The gut microbiota is intimately connected to the immune system, and probiotics like those found in yogurt and supplements can help keep it healthy.

12. Maintain Your Social Links:

Positive effects on mental and emotional health, which in turn boost immune function, have been linked to maintaining social relationships and a solid support system.

13. Consult a Doctor:

• If you have any preexisting illnesses or are worried about your immune system, it is best to seek the advice of a medical practitioner.

While these methods can help keep your immune system strong, they are not a replacement for a well-balanced diet and regular exercise. Combining them with an otherwise healthy lifestyle can do wonders for your immune system. Consult a healthcare expert for individualized guidance if you have specific health issues or illnesses that may impact your immune system.

Children's Tonsillitis

Children between the ages of 5 and 15 are most likely to contract tonsillitis, a common childhood illness. Inflammation of the tonsils, which are two oval-shaped structures in the back of the throat, is the primary symptom of this illness. Children can get tonsillitis from the same viruses and germs that adults get, and the symptoms are generally the same. The following are some important considerations while dealing with pediatric tonsillitis:

1. Causes:

• Viral infections, including rhinovirus, adenovirus, and Epstein-Barr virus (EBV), are the most common causes of tonsillitis in children.

• Strep throat (produced by Group A Streptococcus bacteria) is another prevalent cause of bacterial tonsillitis. Antibiotics are the standard treatment for strep throat.

2. Symptoms:

A painful throat, difficulty swallowing, fever, swollen and red tonsils, headache, and maybe abdominal pain are all symptoms of tonsillitis in youngsters.

Additional symptoms in younger children include drooling, irritability, unwillingness to eat, and restless sleep as a result of pain.

3. Contagiousness:

Tonsillitis, and especially strep throat, is an extremely contagious illness. Transmission can occur through close contact, such as while using the same cutlery or living in the same house as an infected individual.

If you want to stop the transmission of the disease, it's important to teach afflicted kids to cover their mouths and noses when they cough or sneeze and to practice proper hand hygiene yourself.

4. Diagnosis:

Tonsillitis can be diagnosed by a doctor after a thorough physical examination, a throat swab, and sometimes blood testing to rule out other potential causes of the infection.

5. Treatment:

With bed rest, fluids, and over-the-counter pain medications, viral tonsillitis usually goes away on its own.

Antibiotics are necessary for the treatment of bacterial tonsillitis, especially strep throat. Antibiotics should be used for the full duration of treatment.

6. Complications:

Seek medical assistance quickly if your child exhibits symptoms of strep throat; otherwise, they may develop a more serious infection, such as rheumatic fever, if left untreated.

• Tonsillectomy, the surgical removal of the tonsils, may be recommended for children with recurrent or chronic tonsillitis.

7. Prevention:

• Promote excellent hygiene practices in children, including regular handwashing and avoiding close contact with infectious individuals.

• Teach kids to cover their mouths and noses with a tissue or their elbows when they cough or sneeze.

• Get your kiddos up-to-date on all of their vaccines, including flu shots.

Consult a medical professional if your kid develops tonsillitis symptoms, especially if strep throat is suspected. Effective therapy can

help your kid heal more quickly and
lessen the risk of problems.

CHAPTER FIVE
Complications Associated with Childhood Tonsillitis

Untreated or severe tonsillitis in children can cause a number of secondary problems. Bacterial tonsillitis, especially strep throat, is more likely to cause complications than viral tonsillitis. Possible side effects of tonsillitis in kids include the following:

1. Untreated strep throat can lead to the rare but potentially fatal condition known as rheumatic fever. It usually appears after the primary strep infection has cleared up, a few weeks later. Rheumatic fever can damage the heart, joints, skin, and neurological system, resulting to symptoms such as joint pain, fever, and a distinctive skin rash. This illness can result in long-term health consequences, including heart damage.

2. Untreated strep throat can lead to scarlet fever, a streptococcal illness. Symptoms include a red rash that feels like sandpaper and sometimes a high temperature, a sore throat, and what some people call "strawberry tongue."

3. A complication known as a peritonsillar abscess can develop in some patients. It's a localized accumulation of pus near the tonsils that causes swelling in the throat and neck and brings on excruciating discomfort when swallowing and other symptoms. Sometimes, surgical drainage of a peritonsillar abscess is required.

4.Post-streptococcal glomerulonephritis is an inflammatory disorder of the kidneys that can develop in extremely rare cases when strep throat goes untreated. Blood in the urine (hematuria) and edema are possible symptoms.

5. Scar Tissue: Recurrent or severe tonsillitis can lead to the creation of scar tissue on the tonsils, which may result in continued throat difficulties, including trouble swallowing and a persistent painful throat.

6. Snoring and obstructive sleep apnea can be caused by a child's enlarged tonsils, which can occur for a variety of reasons, including but not limited to recurrent tonsillitis.

7. Children who get tonsillitis frequently or severely are at risk for growth and developmental problems because they may have trouble eating and sleeping adequately.

8. Some kids who get tonsillitis a lot may end up with a chronic version of the disease that causes ongoing throat pain and discomfort.

If your child has tonsillitis symptoms, especially if strep throat is also a possibility, immediate medical attention is necessary. A quicker recovery and fewer problems are possible with an early diagnosis and course of antibiotic treatment. Tonsillectomy, the surgical removal of the tonsils, may be recommended by your doctor if your kid develops recurring or severe tonsillitis.

Nutrition and Diet's Impact

Tonsillitis, like many other infections, can be avoided or at least mitigated by taking good care of one's immune system and eating right. A good diet can't make you immune, but it can help your body fight off illness and keep you healthy overall. Here are some ways in which a healthy diet and nutrition can support a robust immune system:

1. Support your immune system with critical nutrients, vitamins, and minerals found in a balanced diet consisting of foods from all food categories. Ensure that your

child's diet includes a mix of fruits, vegetables, whole grains, lean meats, and healthy fats.

2. Minerals and Vitamins:

Citrus fruits, strawberries, and bell peppers are good sources of vitamin C, which is essential for healthy immune system function and aids the body in warding off infections.

Vitamin D, which is essential for immunological function, can be gained from sun exposure and fortified meals.

The immune system benefits from zinc, which may be found in foods like beans, nuts, and lean meats.

• Iron: Iron is crucial for general health and may aid in awarding against anemia, which can lower the body's defenses.

3. Yogurt and kefir are good examples of foods that contain probiotic microorganisms. They support the immune system by keeping the gut flora in good shape.

4. Keeping yourself adequately hydrated is critical to your health. Drinking adequate water helps

preserve mucous membrane health and boosts immunological function.

5. Limit Your Sugar Intake: An overly sweet diet has been shown to suppress the immune system. Restrict your child's consumption of sugary beverages and foods.

6. **Antioxidants:** Antioxidant-rich foods, like nuts, seeds, and dark leafy greens, help shield cells from damage caused by free radicals and boost the immune system.

7. **Omega-3 Fatty Acids**: These can be found in salmon, flaxseeds, and walnuts, and they help reduce

inflammation and maintain a healthy immune system.

8. Whole grains, such as brown rice, quinoa, and whole wheat bread, are beneficial to health because they are high in fiber and contain critical nutrients.

9. Lean protein sources like poultry, fish, and beans are essential for preserving muscle mass and bolstering the immune system.

10. Reduce Your Intake of Processed Foods: Many processed foods are extremely heavy in unhealthy ingredients including salt, sugar, and fat.

11. Although not related to food, vaccines play a critical role in awarding against infectious diseases and should not be overlooked.

A strong immune system relies on many factors, one of which is eating right. It's also important to get enough sleep, exercise regularly, deal with stress well, and maintain decent cleanliness. Supporting your child's health and immunity over time begins with encouraging appropriate food habits from an early age. Consult a doctor or a qualified dietitian for individualized guidance on any nutritional problems or queries you may have.

Conclusion

Inflammation of the tonsils (tonsillitis) is a frequent illness, especially in youngsters. Symptoms include a painful throat, trouble swallowing, and fever and can be caused by either a virus or bacteria. Recognizing the symptoms correctly is critical for getting medical help quickly.

Tonsillitis treatment hinges on identifying and addressing the underlying cause. In most cases, tonsillitis can be treated with rest, fluids, and painkillers if it is caused by a virus; however, antibiotics are usually necessary to treat bacterial tonsillitis, especially strep throat, to prevent complications. Tonsillectomy is an option for those who suffer from chronic or severe tonsillitis.

Preventing tonsillitis and supporting a healthy immune system entail several techniques, including proper hygiene habits, vaccination, having a balanced diet, staying hydrated, getting enough sleep, and controlling stress. While these steps can help lessen the likelihood of contracting tonsillitis and other infections, it's important to keep in mind that they aren't foolproof and that a generally healthy lifestyle is what really helps the immune system thrive.

If you or your kid is experiencing symptoms of tonsillitis, it is important to see a doctor. Getting the right care at the right time can help avoid complications and speed up the healing process.

THE END

67